PLANT-BASED DIET COOKBOOK FOR SENIORS

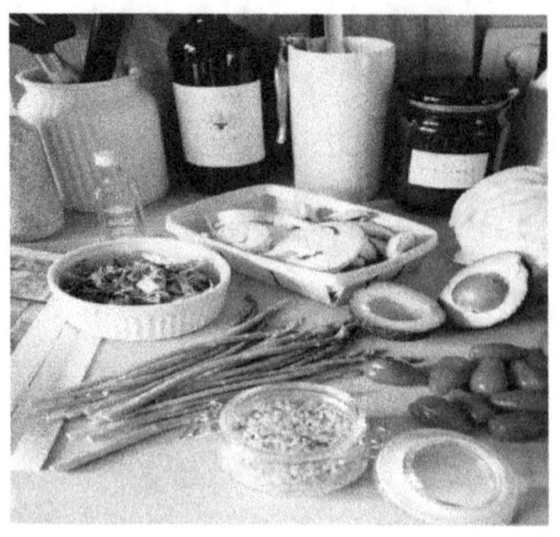

Wholesome Plant-Based Recipes for Vibrant Elder Years

Mary MAY

Table of Contents

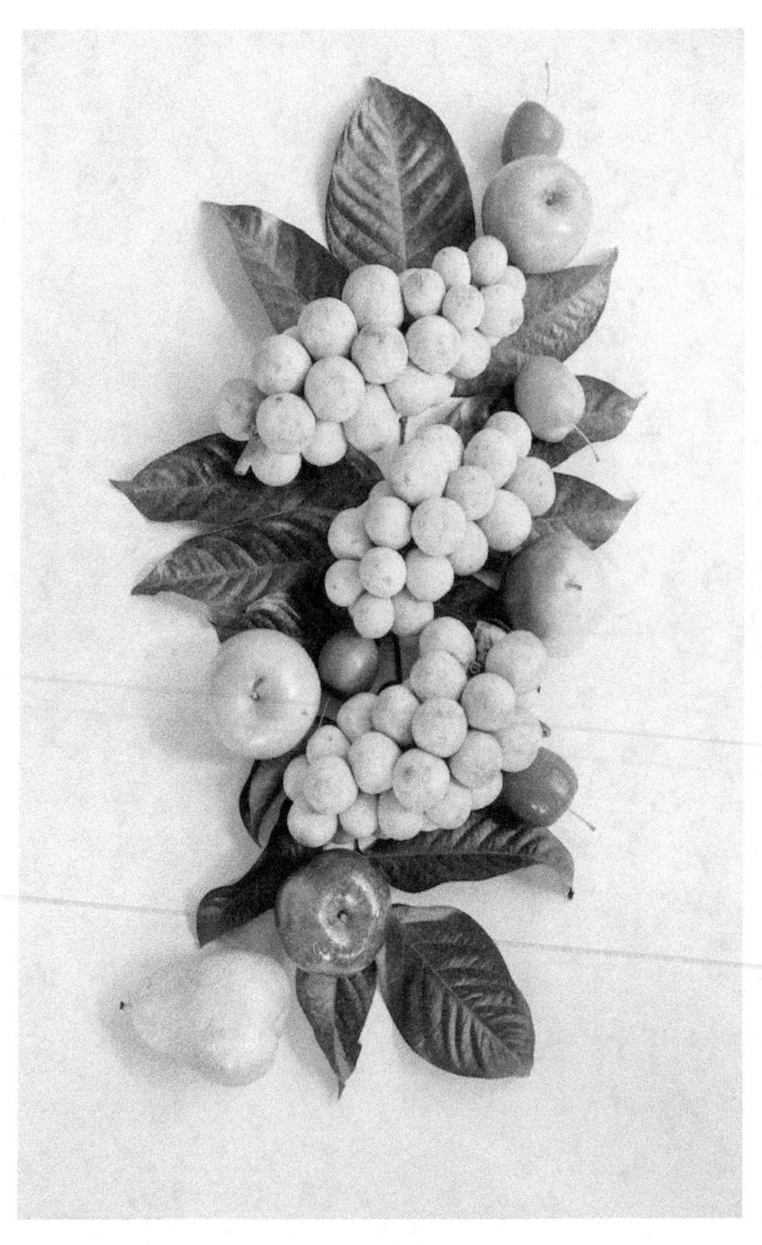

Introduction

Once upon a time in a quiet village, lived an elderly woman named Edith. She had always been passionate about gardening, but as she grew older, she found it harder to maintain her garden. One day, while browsing the shelves of the village library, she stumbled upon a vibrant cookbook titled "The Garden-to-Table Plant-Based Delights."

Intrigued, Edith took the cookbook home and began to flip through its pages. The colorful photographs and detailed recipes inspired her. As she read about the benefits of a plant-based diet, she decided to give it a try. With renewed enthusiasm, she revitalized her garden, dedicating a section to various vegetables, fruits, and herbs.

Edith followed the cookbook's guidance diligently. She planted a variety of tomatoes, leafy greens, peppers, and even experimented with exotic herbs. As the months went by, her garden flourished, and so did her health. She found joy in nurturing her plants and watching them thrive.

The cookbook's recipes became a culinary adventure for Edith. She whipped up dishes like roasted vegetable medleys, hearty lentil soups, and colorful fruit salads. Her friends and neighbors were amazed by her newfound energy and the delicious meals she shared with them.

Word of Edith's transformation spread throughout the village. People started seeking her advice on gardening and cooking. She hosted workshops in her garden, teaching others about the benefits of a plant-based diet and how to grow their own produce. The community came together, inspired by her passion and knowledge.

As seasons changed, so did Edith's garden. It transformed into a lush haven of flavors and colors, showcasing the beauty and bounty of nature. With her radiant health and newfound purpose, Edith proved that age was just a number. Her journey from discovering the cookbook to transforming her life and community through plant-based goodness became an inspiring tale passed down for generations.

Embrace the transformative power of age with "Nourishing Wisdom: A Plant-Based Diet Cookbook for Elders." This culinary journey is a celebration of vitality and well-being, curated specifically for those embracing their golden years. Drawing inspiration from the bountiful offerings of nature, this cookbook serves as your guide to a vibrant and fulfilling life through the art of plant-based eating.

In these pages, you will discover a harmonious fusion of flavors, nutrients, and culinary traditions carefully tailored to meet the unique nutritional needs of seniors. From hearty breakfasts that kickstart your day to delectable dinners that ignite the senses, each recipe has been thoughtfully crafted to nourish the body and invigorate the spirit.

"Nourishing Wisdom" isn't just a collection of recipes; it's a holistic approach to wellness that honors the wisdom gained over a lifetime. With insights into the benefits of a plant-based diet on cognitive function, heart health, and overall vitality, this cookbook empowers elders to make informed choices that resonate with their well-being goals.

Whether you're a seasoned plant-based enthusiast or someone exploring this dietary path for the first time, "Nourishing Wisdom" offers a treasure trove of culinary inspiration, practical tips for meal preparation, and a roadmap for embracing the joy of mindful eating. As you embark on this flavorful journey, may you discover the joy of savoring delicious meals that not only nurture your body but also nourish your soul. Welcome to a world where age is an opportunity to thrive, and each meal is a step towards a future brimming with health and happiness.

Chapter One: The Basics of Plant-Based Nutrition

Plant-based nutrition centers around consuming a variety of plant foods such as fruits, vegetables, grains, legumes, nuts, and seeds. This approach avoids or limits the intake of animal products like meat, dairy, eggs, and other animal-derived ingredients.

Benefits of Plant-Based Nutrition

1. **Improved Heart Health:** Plant-based diets are associated with lower cholesterol levels, blood pressure, and reduced risk of heart diseases.

2. **Weight Management:** Plant-based diets are often lower in calories and saturated fats, making them beneficial for weight loss and maintenance.

3. **Lower Risk of Chronic Diseases:** Studies suggest that plant-based diets may lower the risk of type 2 diabetes, certain cancers, and obesity-related diseases.

4. **Digestive Health:** High fiber content in plant foods promotes healthy digestion and can prevent constipation.

5. **Environmental Sustainability:** Plant-based diets have a lower carbon footprint and contribute to reducing greenhouse gas emissions.

6. **Ethical Considerations:** Many people adopt plant-based diets to align their eating habits with animal welfare concerns.

Key Nutrients in Plant-Based Diets

1. **Protein:** Sources include legumes (beans, lentils, chickpeas), tofu, tempeh, nuts, seeds, and whole grains.

2. **Iron:** Found in lentils, beans, fortified cereals, spinach, and quinoa. Pairing iron-rich foods with vitamin C enhances absorption.

3. **Calcium:** Besides dairy, calcium sources include fortified plant milks, leafy greens (kale, broccoli), tofu, and almonds.

4. **Vitamin B12:** Essential for nerve function, it's mainly found in animal products, so B12-fortified foods or supplements are recommended.

5. **Omega-3 Fatty Acids:** Flaxseeds, chia seeds, walnuts, and algae-based supplements provide essential fatty acids.

6. **Vitamin D:** Fortified plant milks and exposure to sunlight can help meet vitamin D needs.

7. **Zinc:** Beans, nuts, seeds, and whole grains are good sources of zinc in plant-based diets.

Tips for a Balanced Plant-Based Diet

1. **Variety:** Consume a diverse range of fruits, vegetables, grains, legumes, nuts, and seeds to ensure a broad spectrum of nutrients.

2. **Whole Foods:** Opt for minimally processed foods over heavily refined options.

3. **Protein Combinations:** Pair different plant protein sources (beans with rice, hummus with whole wheat pita) to ensure complete amino acid profiles.

4. **Healthy Fats:** Incorporate sources of healthy fats like avocados, nuts, and seeds.

5. **Supplements:** Consider vitamin B12 and, if necessary, vitamin D and omega-3 supplements.

6. **Read Labels:** Be mindful of hidden animal-derived ingredients in packaged foods.

7. **Plan Meals:** Plan balanced meals in advance to ensure you're meeting your nutritional needs.

Understanding the Plant-Based Diet

In an era where dietary choices have profound implications for personal health, environmental sustainability, and ethical considerations, the concept of a plant-based diet has gained substantial prominence. Rooted in the fundamental principle of prioritizing plant-derived foods while minimizing or eliminating animal products, the plant-based diet represents a holistic approach to nourishment that transcends individual plates.

Foundations of a Plant-Based Diet

At its essence, a plant-based diet is centered around consuming a wide array of foods derived from plants. This includes fruits, vegetables, whole grains, legumes (beans, lentils, peas), nuts, seeds, and plant-based oils. The goal is to harness the abundant nutritional benefits found in these foods, ranging from essential vitamins and minerals to dietary fiber and antioxidants.

Diversity and Flexibility

The beauty of the plant-based diet lies in its adaptability. It's not a rigid template but rather a spectrum of dietary choices that accommodate individual preferences and needs. This spectrum ranges from strict vegans – who eliminate all animal products – to vegetarians who might still consume dairy or eggs. Flexitarians or those who are simply reducing their meat intake also fall within this spectrum. This flexibility encourages a gradual transition towards more plant-centered choices.

Nutrient Profile of Plant-Based Foods

Plant-based foods provide an array of essential nutrients that are key to maintaining optimal health:

1. **Proteins:** Contrary to misconceptions, plant sources offer ample protein. Legumes, tofu, tempeh, seitan, quinoa, and nuts are all rich in protein, supporting muscle growth and repair.

2. **Fiber:** Whole plant foods are abundant in dietary fiber, promoting digestive health, regulating blood sugar levels, and providing a sense of satiety.

3. **Vitamins and Minerals:** Fruits and vegetables are brimming with vitamins like vitamin C, vitamin A, and various B vitamins, as well as minerals like potassium, magnesium, and calcium.

4. **Healthy Fats:** Nuts, seeds, avocados, and plant-based oils provide essential fatty acids that support heart health and cognitive function.

Health Benefits of a Plant-Based Diet

Numerous studies have indicated the potential health benefits associated with adopting a plant-based diet:

1. **Cardiovascular Health:** The reduced intake of saturated fats found in animal products and the increased consumption of fiber-rich plants can contribute to a healthier heart.

2. **Weight Management:** Plant-based diets are often lower in calorie density and higher in fiber, making them conducive to weight management and satiety.

3. **Diabetes Management:** Plant-based diets can help improve insulin sensitivity and manage blood sugar levels.

4. **Lower Risk of Chronic Diseases:** Regular consumption of fruits, vegetables, and whole grains is linked to a reduced risk of chronic diseases such

as type 2 diabetes, certain cancers, and hypertension.

Ethical and Environmental Considerations

Beyond personal health, adopting a plant-based diet aligns with broader ethical and environmental considerations:

1. **Animal Welfare:** By reducing or eliminating animal products, individuals can actively contribute to the reduction of animal suffering in industrial farming practices.

2. **Environmental Impact:** Plant-based diets have a lower carbon footprint, requiring less land, water, and resources compared to animal-based diets. This helps mitigate deforestation, water pollution, and greenhouse gas emissions.

Embracing the Plant-Based Lifestyle

Transitioning to a plant-based diet requires mindful planning and informed choices:

1. **Balanced Diet:** Focus on variety, incorporating different colors, textures, and types of plant foods to ensure a well-rounded nutrient intake.

2. **Protein Diversity:** Explore various plant protein sources to ensure adequate intake of essential amino acids.

3. **Supplementation:** Consider vitamin B12 supplementation, as it's primarily found in animal products.

4. **Gradual Transition:** Ease into the plant-based lifestyle, making gradual changes to allow your palate and body to adapt.

Nutritional Needs of Seniors on a Plant-Based Diet

As individuals age, their nutritional needs evolve, requiring careful consideration to ensure optimal health and well-being. A plant-based diet can offer numerous benefits for seniors, including reduced risk of chronic diseases, improved digestion, and enhanced vitality. However, it's essential to tailor this diet to meet the unique nutritional requirements of older adults. This comprehensive guide explores the nutritional needs of seniors on a plant-based diet, offering insights into key nutrients, meal planning, and practical tips for maintaining health in the golden years.

Key Nutrients for Seniors on a Plant-Based Diet

1. **Protein:** Adequate protein intake is crucial for maintaining muscle mass and preventing sarcopenia, a condition

characterized by the loss of muscle tissue. Sources of plant-based protein include legumes (beans, lentils, chickpeas), tofu, tempeh, seitan, nuts, seeds, and whole grains.

2. **Calcium and Vitamin D:** Seniors need sufficient calcium for bone health, and vitamin D facilitates calcium absorption. Plant-based calcium sources include fortified plant milk, fortified orange juice, leafy greens (kale, collard greens, bok choy), almonds, and chia seeds. Vitamin D can be obtained through sunlight exposure and fortified foods.

3. **B Vitamins:** Vitamin B12 is especially important for seniors as its absorption tends to decrease with age. Fortified foods like cereals, plant milk, and nutritional yeast can provide this vital nutrient. B vitamins are also found in whole grains, legumes, and leafy greens.

4. **Omega-3 Fatty Acids:** These fats support heart and brain health. Seniors can obtain omega-3s from flaxseeds, chia seeds, walnuts, hemp seeds, and algae-based supplements.

5. **Fiber:** Fiber aids digestion, regulates blood sugar, and supports a healthy gut. Whole plant foods like fruits, vegetables, whole grains, legumes, and seeds are excellent sources of dietary fiber.

6. **Iron:** Plant-based iron sources include lentils, beans, tofu, spinach, quinoa, fortified cereals, and pumpkin seeds. Consuming vitamin C-rich foods alongside iron-rich foods enhances iron absorption.

Meal Planning and Practical Tips

1. **Variety is Key:** Seniors should aim for a diverse range of plant foods to ensure they obtain a wide spectrum of nutrients.

2. **Portion Control:** Older adults typically have lower calorie needs, so portion control is vital to prevent overeating. Focus on nutrient-dense foods.

3. **Hydration:** Adequate hydration becomes more critical with age. Encourage drinking water, herbal teas, and consuming water-rich foods like fruits and vegetables.

4. **Snacking:** Opt for healthy snacks like nuts, seeds, fruits, vegetables, and whole-grain crackers to maintain energy levels between meals.

5. **Supplements:** Consult a healthcare professional to determine if supplements like B12, vitamin D, or omega-3s are necessary.

6. **Cooking Techniques:** Choose cooking methods that preserve nutrients, such as steaming, baking, roasting, and sautéing, while minimizing deep frying.

7. **Social Engagement:** Eating meals with friends or family can improve the dining experience and enhance nutrient absorption through better digestion.

8. **Regular Health Check-ups:** Seniors should schedule regular check-ups to monitor nutrient levels and overall health.

Exploring Essential Nutrients: Protein, Calcium, Vitamin D, B12, and More

Proper nutrition is the foundation of a healthy lifestyle, providing the body with the essential components it needs to function optimally. Essential nutrients are substances that the body cannot produce on its own and must be obtained from the diet. Among these vital nutrients, protein, calcium, vitamin D, vitamin B12, and others play pivotal roles in maintaining overall health, supporting bodily functions, and preventing various health issues. This article delves into the significance, sources, and benefits of these essential nutrients.

1. Protein: *Building Blocks of Life*

Proteins are the fundamental building blocks of the body. They are composed of amino acids, which play critical roles in repairing tissues, building muscles, supporting immune function, and producing enzymes and hormones. Dietary protein sources include lean meats, poultry, fish, eggs, dairy products, legumes, nuts, and seeds. Adequate protein intake is especially important for individuals engaged in physical activities, as it aids in muscle recovery and growth.

2. Calcium: *Strong Bones and Beyond*

Calcium is renowned for its role in promoting strong bones and teeth. It is also essential for proper muscle function, nerve transmission, and blood clotting. Dairy products like milk, yogurt, and cheese are well-known sources of calcium. Additionally, dark leafy greens, fortified plant-based milk, and almonds provide non-dairy options for obtaining this vital nutrient.

3. Vitamin D: *The Sunshine Vitamin*

Vitamin D is crucial for calcium absorption and bone health. It also contributes to immune system function, cell growth, and inflammation regulation. The skin produces vitamin D when

exposed to sunlight, and dietary sources include fatty fish (salmon, mackerel), fortified dairy and plant-based milk, egg yolks, and supplements.

4. Vitamin B12: *Nervous System Support*

Vitamin B12 is essential for maintaining a healthy nervous system, forming red blood cells, and aiding in DNA synthesis. It is predominantly found in animal products such as meat, fish, eggs, and dairy. Vegans and vegetarians should ensure they obtain sufficient B12 through fortified foods or supplements.

5. Iron: *Oxygen Transport and Energy Production*

Iron is critical for oxygen transport in the blood and energy production within cells. Heme iron, found in animal products, is more readily absorbed than non-heme iron from plant sources. Foods like red meat, poultry, lentils, spinach, and fortified cereals are good sources of iron.

6. Folate (Vitamin B9): *Cell Growth and Development*

Folate is essential for cell growth and development, particularly during pregnancy when it helps prevent birth defects. Leafy greens, legumes, fortified grains, and citrus fruits are excellent sources of folate.

7. Fiber: *Digestive Health*

While not a nutrient in the traditional sense, dietary fiber is vital for digestive health. It aids in regulating bowel movements, maintaining gut health, and preventing constipation. Whole grains, fruits, vegetables, nuts, and seeds are rich sources of dietary fiber.

8. Omega-3 Fatty Acids: *Heart and Brain Health*

Omega-3 fatty acids are renowned for their heart-protective and brain-boosting benefits. They help reduce inflammation, support cardiovascular health, and contribute to brain function. Fatty fish (salmon, sardines),

flaxseeds, chia seeds, and walnuts are excellent sources of omega-3s.

9. Potassium: *Electrolyte Balance*

Potassium is an electrolyte that helps maintain fluid and electrolyte balance, nerve function, and muscle contractions. Bananas, potatoes, leafy greens, and beans are rich sources of potassium.

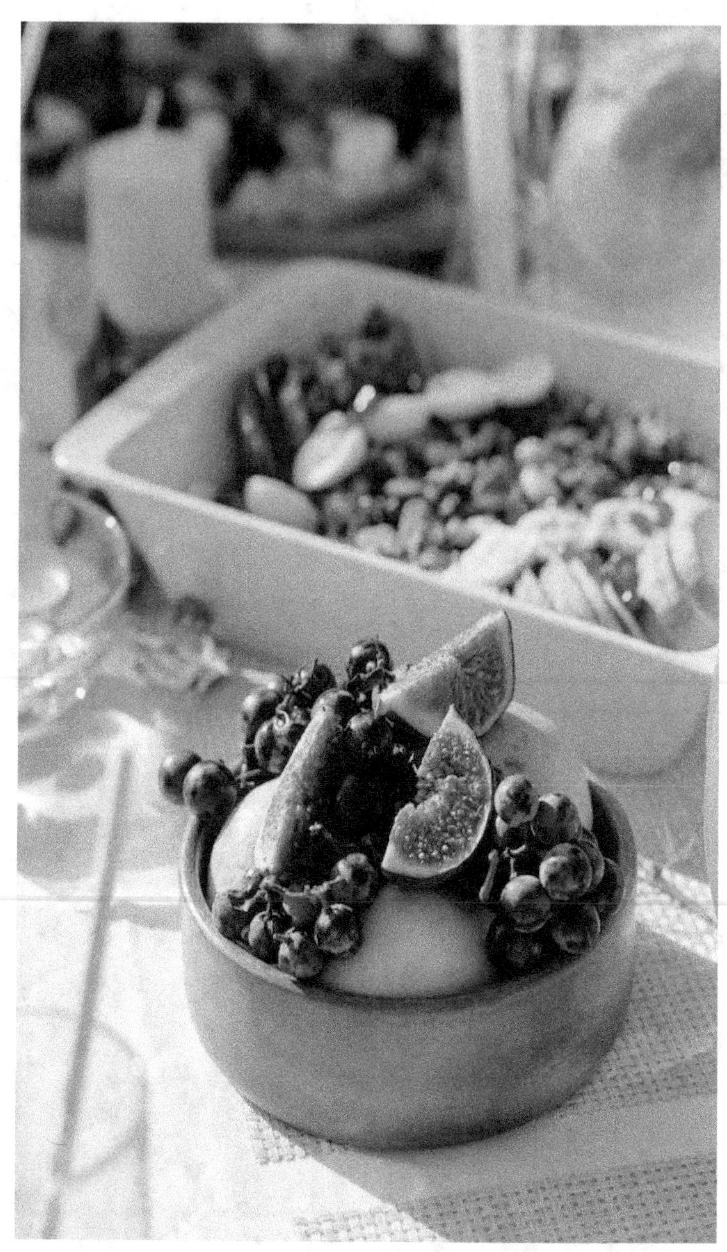

Chapter Two: Planning Wholesome Plant-Based Meals

Plant-based diets have gained widespread attention for their numerous health benefits and positive impacts on the environment. A well-planned plant-based meal can provide all the essential nutrients your body needs while promoting overall well-being. Whether you're a seasoned vegan or just starting to explore plant-based eating, understanding the principles of planning wholesome plant-based meals is essential to ensure you're getting the nutrients you need. Here's a comprehensive guide to help you plan nutritious and delicious plant-based meals:

1. Diverse Nutrient Intake:

A key principle of any balanced diet, including plant-based, is to consume a variety of nutrients. Make sure to include a wide range of fruits, vegetables, whole grains, legumes, nuts, and seeds in your meals. Each food group contributes different vitamins, minerals, fiber, and antioxidants essential for your health.

2. Protein Sources:

Plant-based protein sources include beans, lentils, chickpeas, tofu, tempeh, quinoa, nuts, and seeds. Combining different protein sources in a meal can enhance the quality of protein intake and provide all essential amino acids. Aim to include protein-rich foods in every meal to support muscle health and overall satiety.

3. Whole Grains:

Whole grains like brown rice, quinoa, whole wheat pasta, and oats are excellent sources of complex carbohydrates and fiber. They provide sustained energy and promote digestive health. Choose whole grains over refined grains to ensure you're benefiting from the complete nutritional profile of the grain.

4. Healthy Fats:

Include sources of healthy fats in your meals such as avocados, nuts, seeds, and olive oil. These fats are important for brain health, hormone production, and overall cell function. Remember to consume these fats in moderation, as they are calorie-dense.

5. Calcium and Vitamin D:

Dairy products are often a significant source of calcium and vitamin D, but there are plant-based alternatives available. Fortified plant-based milk (such as almond, soy, or oat milk) and leafy green vegetables (like kale and collard greens) can help meet your calcium needs. Vitamin D can be obtained from sunlight exposure or fortified foods.

6. Iron and Vitamin B12:

Iron is important for oxygen transport in the blood, and vitamin B12 is crucial for nerve function and red blood cell production. Plant-based iron sources include beans, lentils, spinach, and fortified cereals. However, plant-based iron is non-heme iron, which is less efficiently absorbed. Pairing iron-rich foods with vitamin C-rich foods (like citrus fruits) can enhance absorption. For vitamin B12, consider fortified foods or supplements, as it's primarily found in animal products.

7. Omega-3 Fatty Acids:

Omega-3 fatty acids are important for heart and brain health. Include flaxseeds, chia seeds, walnuts, and hemp seeds in your meals to obtain plant-based sources of omega-3s. If necessary, consider an algae-based omega-3 supplement.

8. Plan Balanced Meals:

A balanced plant-based meal should include:

- A source of protein (beans, lentils, tofu, etc.).
- A variety of colorful vegetables and leafy greens.
- Whole grains or starchy vegetables for carbohydrates.

- Healthy fats from nuts, seeds, or avocados.
- Flavorful herbs, spices, and seasonings to enhance taste.

9. Meal Prepping:

Meal prepping can simplify plant-based eating. Prepare staples like grains, legumes, and chopped vegetables in advance. This makes it easier to assemble nutritious meals throughout the week, especially on busy days.

10. Listen to Your Body:

Everyone's nutritional needs are different. Pay attention to how your body responds to different foods and adjust your diet accordingly. If needed, consult a registered dietitian or nutritionist to ensure you're meeting your nutrient requirements.

Crafting Balanced Meals for Optimal Nutrition

A balanced meal is the cornerstone of a healthy lifestyle, providing the body with the essential nutrients it needs to function at its best. Crafting balanced meals involves carefully selecting a variety of nutrient-rich foods that fulfill the body's requirements for energy, vitamins, minerals, protein, carbohydrates, and healthy fats. This comprehensive guide explores the key principles of crafting balanced meals to achieve optimal nutrition.

Understanding the Components of Balanced Meals

1. Protein:

Protein is vital for tissue repair, immune function, and muscle development. Include sources such as lean meats, poultry, fish, eggs, dairy products, legumes, and plant-based alternatives like tofu and tempeh.

2. Carbohydrates:

Carbohydrates provide energy and should come from whole grains (brown rice, quinoa, whole wheat), starchy vegetables (sweet potatoes, corn), and fruits. Prioritize complex carbohydrates over refined options.

3. Healthy Fats:

Healthy fats support brain health, hormone production, and overall wellbeing. Incorporate sources like avocados, nuts, seeds, olive oil, and fatty fish (salmon, mackerel) rich in omega-3 fatty acids.

4. Vegetables:

Colorful and non-starchy vegetables provide vitamins, minerals, antioxidants, and fiber. Aim to fill half your plate with vegetables, including leafy greens, broccoli, peppers, and carrots.

5.   Fruits:

Fruits offer natural sugars, vitamins, and fiber. Opt for a variety of fresh, whole fruits to satisfy your sweet cravings and boost nutrient intake.

The Plate Method

The plate method is a visual guide that simplifies the process of crafting balanced meals. Divide your plate into four sections:

1. **Vegetables:** Fill half your plate with a variety of colorful vegetables.
2. **Protein:** Allocate a quarter of your plate to lean proteins like chicken, fish, tofu, or beans.
3. **Carbohydrates:** Reserve the remaining quarter for whole grains or starchy vegetables.
4. **Side:** Include a small portion of healthy fats or dairy on the side.

Portion Control

Balanced meals also require proper portion control to avoid overeating and maintain a healthy weight. Using smaller plates and paying attention to hunger and fullness cues can help you regulate portion sizes.

Nutrient-Dense Choices

Opt for nutrient-dense foods that pack a high nutritional punch for their calorie content. Examples include leafy greens, berries, nuts, seeds, lean proteins, and whole grains.

Hydration

Water is essential for digestion, circulation, and overall bodily functions. Drink water throughout the day and limit sugary beverages.

Meal Planning

Plan your meals and snacks ahead of time to ensure you have a variety of nutrient-rich foods available. This can help you avoid last-minute unhealthy choices.

Special Considerations

1. **Dietary Restrictions:** Tailor your balanced meals to accommodate any dietary restrictions or allergies you may have.

2. **Health Goals:** Adjust your meal composition based on your health goals, whether it's weight loss, muscle gain, or managing a specific health condition.

3. **Lifestyle:** Consider your lifestyle and activity level when determining your caloric needs and portion sizes.

Meal Prepping and Batch Cooking for Seniors

As individuals age, their dietary needs and cooking abilities can change. Meal prepping and batch cooking are effective strategies that can significantly benefit seniors in maintaining a healthy and convenient eating routine. In this comprehensive guide, we will explore the advantages of meal prepping and batch cooking for seniors, along with practical tips to implement these strategies successfully.

Benefits of Meal Prepping and Batch Cooking for Seniors

1. Nutritional Health:

Maintaining proper nutrition becomes even more crucial as people age. Meal prepping and batch cooking enable seniors to plan and prepare balanced meals that meet their specific nutritional requirements. This approach ensures that they receive essential vitamins, minerals, and macronutrients necessary for overall health and wellbeing.

2. Time and Energy Efficiency:

Preparing meals daily can be time-consuming and draining, especially for seniors with limited energy. Meal prepping and batch cooking involve cooking larger quantities of food at once and portioning them for future consumption. This saves time and energy throughout the week, allowing seniors to focus on other activities they enjoy.

3. Consistency in Diet:

Seniors often face challenges in adhering to a consistent diet due to factors such as limited mobility or cognitive changes. Meal prepping and batch cooking establish a routine, making it easier for seniors to stick to their dietary plans and avoid relying on less nutritious convenience foods.

4. Cost Savings:

Buying ingredients in bulk for batch cooking can lead to cost savings. Seniors can take advantage of sales, discounts, and reduced packaging, thus optimizing their food budget. Additionally, by planning meals ahead, there's less likelihood of purchasing unnecessary items or letting ingredients go to waste.

5. Portion Control:

Maintaining a healthy weight and preventing overeating is essential for seniors. Meal prepping involves portioning meals in advance, which helps seniors manage their caloric intake and avoid overindulgence. This controlled approach to eating can contribute to weight management and overall health.

6. Independence:

Seniors who live alone or have limited access to support may find meal prepping and batch cooking invaluable for maintaining their independence. By having nutritious, pre-prepared meals, seniors can avoid the challenges of daily cooking while still enjoying home-cooked meals.

Practical Tips for Successful Meal Prepping and Batch Cooking

1. Plan Your Meals:

Create a weekly meal plan that includes breakfast, lunch, dinner, and snacks. Consider incorporating a variety of foods from different food groups to ensure a balanced diet. Make note of any dietary restrictions or preferences when planning your meals.

2. Choose Seniors-Friendly Recipes:

Opt for recipes that are simple, with minimal ingredients and straightforward cooking techniques. Look for recipes that can be adapted to larger batches without compromising taste or quality. Slow cooker meals, one-pan dishes, and casseroles are excellent options.

3. Make a Shopping List:

Based on your meal plan, create a detailed shopping list of the ingredients you'll need. Stick to your list to avoid purchasing unnecessary items. Shopping with a list can also help streamline the grocery shopping process.

4. Prep in Batches:

Designate a specific day or time for batch cooking. Cook larger quantities of proteins, grains, and vegetables that can be used across different meals. Once cooked, portion these components into individual containers for easy access.

5. Invest in Storage Containers:

Invest in high-quality, airtight storage containers that are microwave and freezer safe. Clear containers are especially useful, allowing you to easily identify the contents and monitor freshness.

6. Label and Date:

Label each container with the meal's name and date of preparation. This ensures that you use meals before they expire and helps you keep track of your inventory.

7. Freeze with Care:

If you've prepared more meals than you can consume within a few days, consider freezing them for later use. Properly wrap and seal items to prevent freezer burn. Soups, stews, and sauces freeze particularly well.

8. Reheating Instructions:

Include reheating instructions on your labeled containers. This makes it simple to enjoy your prepped meals without any guesswork.

9. Hydration Matters:

Don't forget to include beverages in your meal prep routine. Prepare infused water, herbal teas, or other hydrating options to stay refreshed throughout the day.

10. Rotate and Modify:

To prevent meal fatigue, rotate through a variety of recipes and modify ingredients to keep things interesting. This approach ensures that you continue to enjoy your meals and receive a range of nutrients.

A Week's Worth of Plant-Based Meal Plans

Embracing a plant-based diet has gained immense popularity in recent years due to its health benefits, positive environmental impact, and ethical considerations. A well-planned plant-based meal plan can provide all the essential nutrients while catering to diverse tastes and preferences. In this guide, we present a comprehensive week's worth of plant-based meal plans that offer variety, balance, and deliciousness.

Day 1: Energizing Start

Breakfast:

- Creamy oatmeal topped with mixed berries, chopped nuts, and a drizzle of almond butter.

Lunch:

- Chickpea and vegetable stir-fry with quinoa, seasoned with ginger, garlic, and tamari.

Dinner:

- Lentil and vegetable curry served with brown rice and a side of steamed broccoli.

Day 2: Fresh and Light

Breakfast:

- Smoothie bowl with spinach, banana, frozen berries, almond milk, and a sprinkle of chia seeds.

Lunch:

- Mediterranean-inspired salad with mixed greens, cherry tomatoes, cucumbers, olives, red onion, and a balsamic vinaigrette.

Dinner:

- Zucchini noodles tossed in a pesto sauce made from basil, pine nuts, garlic, olive oil, and nutritional yeast.

<u>**Day 3: Hearty Comfort**</u>

Breakfast:

- Whole-grain toast topped with smashed avocado, sliced tomatoes, and a sprinkle of nutritional yeast.

Lunch:

- Three-bean chili served with a side of whole-grain bread or cornbread.

Dinner:

- Stuffed bell peppers filled with a mix of quinoa, black beans, corn, tomatoes, and spices.

<u>**Day 4: Global Flavors**</u>

Breakfast:

- Vegan yogurt parfait layered with granola, diced mango, and a drizzle of agave syrup.

Lunch:

- Thai-inspired peanut noodle salad with rice noodles, colorful vegetables, tofu, and a zesty peanut dressing.

Dinner:

- Mexican-style fajita bowl with sautéed peppers, onions, black beans, salsa, guacamole, and brown rice.

Day 5: Protein-Packed

Breakfast:

- High-protein smoothie with silken tofu, banana, spinach, almond milk, and a spoonful of nut butter.

Lunch:

- Quinoa and black bean salad with roasted sweet potatoes, red cabbage, and a tahini-lime dressing.

Dinner:

- Baked falafel served in whole-grain pita pockets with hummus, shredded lettuce, and cucumber-tomato salad.

Day 6: Wholesome Indulgence

Breakfast:

- Overnight chia pudding made with almond milk, topped with sliced almonds and mixed fruits.

Lunch:

- Vegan chickpea "tuna" salad sandwich with lettuce, tomato, and whole-grain bread.

Dinner:

- Portobello mushroom steaks marinated in balsamic vinegar, grilled and served with quinoa pilaf and steamed asparagus.

Day 7: Nourishing Fare

Breakfast:

- Acai bowl with coconut flakes, banana slices, and a handful of pumpkin seeds.

Lunch:

- Roasted vegetable and hummus wrap in a whole-grain tortilla, with a side of carrot sticks.

Dinner:

- Roasted root vegetables (sweet potatoes, carrots, beets) alongside a kale and citrus salad, drizzled with a lemon-tahini dressing.

Snack Ideas (Throughout the Week)

- Apple slices with almond butter.
- Mixed nuts and seeds.
- Rice cakes topped with avocado and cherry tomatoes.
- Fresh fruit salad.
- Edamame pods sprinkled with sea salt.
- Homemade trail mix with dried fruits and dark chocolate chips.

Chapter Three: Breakfast Delights

Oatmeal with Berries

Ingredients:

- 1/2 cup rolled oats
- 1 cup almond milk (or any plant-based milk)
- 1/2 cup mixed berries (blueberries, strawberries, raspberries)
- 1 tablespoon chopped nuts (almonds, walnuts)
- 1 teaspoon maple syrup (optional)

Instructions:

1. In a saucepan, combine oats and almond milk. Cook over medium heat, stirring occasionally, until the oats are creamy and tender.

2. Top the oatmeal with mixed berries and
    chopped nuts.

3. Drizzle with maple syrup if desired.

Smoothie Bowl

Ingredients:

- 1 ripe banana, frozen
- 1/2 cup frozen mango chunks
- 1/2 cup spinach leaves
- 1/2 cup almond milk
- Toppings: sliced banana, granola, chia seeds

Instructions:

1. Blend frozen banana, frozen mango, spinach, and almond milk until smooth.
2. Pour the smoothie into a bowl and top with sliced banana, granola, and chia seeds.

Chia Seed Pudding

Ingredients:

- 3 tablespoons chia seeds
- 1 cup almond milk
- 1 teaspoon vanilla extract
- Fresh fruit for topping

Instructions:

1. Mix chia seeds, almond milk, and vanilla extract in a bowl.
2. Stir well and let it sit in the refrigerator for at least 2 hours or overnight.
3. Top with fresh fruit before serving.

Vegan Pancakes

Ingredients:

- 1 cup flour (whole wheat or oat flour)
- 1 tablespoon baking powder
- 1 tablespoon sugar (or a natural sweetener)
- 1 cup plant-based milk
- 1 teaspoon vanilla extract

Instructions:

1. In a bowl, whisk together flour, baking powder, and sugar.
2. Add plant-based milk and vanilla extract, and mix until just combined.
3. Heat a non-stick skillet over medium heat. Pour batter to make pancakes and cook until bubbles form on the surface. Flip and cook until golden brown.

Tofu Scramble

Ingredients:

- 1/2 block firm tofu, crumbled
- 1/4 cup diced bell peppers
- 1/4 cup diced tomatoes
- 1/4 cup chopped spinach
- 1/4 teaspoon turmeric
- Salt and pepper to taste

Instructions:

1. In a skillet, sauté bell peppers and tomatoes until soft.
2. Add crumbled tofu and turmeric. Cook for a few minutes, stirring occasionally.
3. Add chopped spinach and cook until wilted. Season with salt and pepper.

Fruit Salad

Ingredients:

- Assorted fresh fruits (bananas, apples, oranges, grapes, etc.)
- Chopped nuts or seeds (almonds, walnuts, pumpkin seeds)

Instructions:

1. Wash, peel, and chop the fruits into bite-sized pieces.
2. Combine the fruits in a bowl and sprinkle with chopped nuts or seeds.

Avocado Toast

Ingredients:

- 1 ripe avocado
- Whole grain bread slices
- Lemon juice
- Red pepper flakes (optional)
- Salt and pepper to taste

Instructions:

1. Mash the avocado in a bowl and add a squeeze of lemon juice, red pepper flakes, salt, and pepper.
2. Toast the bread slices and spread the avocado mixture on top.

Whole Grain Porridge

Ingredients:

- 1/2 cup quinoa or millet
- 1.5 cups water or plant-based milk
- Chopped dried fruits (dates, apricots)
- Cinnamon and nutmeg to taste

Instructions:

1. Rinse quinoa or millet and combine with water or plant-based milk in a saucepan.

2. Cook over medium heat until grains are soft and liquid is absorbed.

3. Stir in chopped dried fruits, cinnamon, and nutmeg.

Nut Butter Banana Wrap

Ingredients:

- Whole grain tortilla or wrap
- Nut butter (almond, peanut, or cashew)
- Sliced banana
- Cinnamon

Instructions:

1. Spread nut butter on the tortilla.
2. Place sliced banana in the center and sprinkle with cinnamon.
3. Roll up the tortilla and slice into smaller pieces if desired.

Coconut Yogurt Parfait

Ingredients:

- Plant-based coconut yogurt
- Mixed berries
- Granola
- Drizzle of agave syrup

Instructions:

1. Layer coconut yogurt, mixed berries, and granola in a glass or bowl.
2. Drizzle with agave syrup for added sweetness.

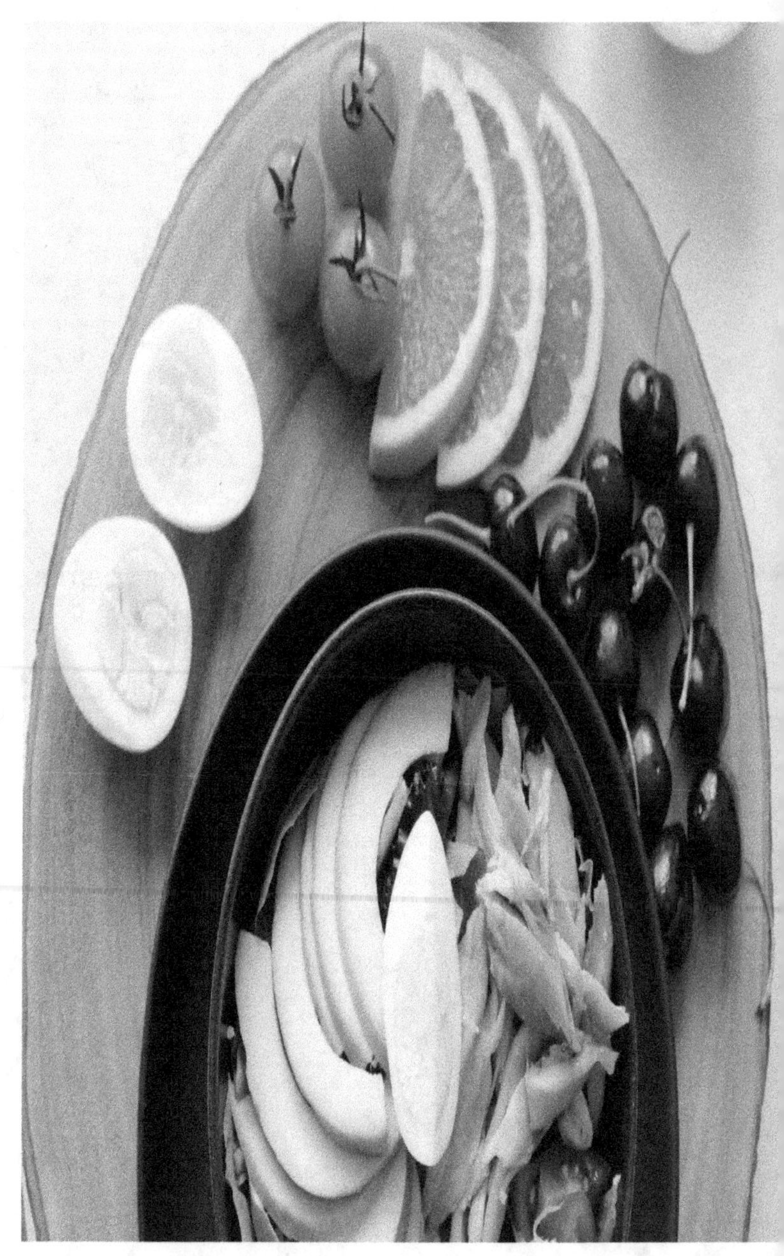

Chapter 4: Lunch

Lentil Soup

Ingredients:

- 1 cup dried green or brown lentils
- 4 cups vegetable broth
- 1 onion, chopped
- 2 carrots, chopped
- 2 celery stalks, chopped
- 2 cloves garlic, minced
- 1 teaspoon cumin
- 1 teaspoon turmeric
- Salt and pepper to taste

Instructions:

1. Rinse lentils and set aside.
2. In a large pot, sauté onions, carrots, and celery until softened.
3. Add garlic, cumin, turmeric, and lentils. Stir to combine.

4. Pour in vegetable broth, bring to a boil, then reduce heat and simmer for about 20-25 minutes until lentils are tender.
5. Season with salt and pepper. Serve hot.

Chickpea Salad

Ingredients:

- 2 cups cooked chickpeas
- 1 cucumber, diced
- 1 red bell pepper, diced
- 1/4 red onion, finely chopped
- 1/4 cup chopped parsley
- Juice of 1 lemon
- 2 tablespoons olive oil
- Salt and pepper to taste

Instructions:

1. In a large bowl, combine chickpeas, cucumber, bell pepper, red onion, and parsley.
2. In a small bowl, whisk together lemon juice, olive oil, salt, and pepper.
3. Pour the dressing over the salad and toss to combine. Serve chilled.

Quinoa Salad

Ingredients:

- 1 cup cooked quinoa
- 1 cup diced mixed vegetables (tomatoes, cucumbers, bell peppers, etc.)
- 1/4 cup chopped fresh herbs (parsley, mint, basil)
- 1/4 cup chopped nuts (walnuts, almonds)
- Lemon vinaigrette (2 tablespoons lemon juice, 2 tablespoons olive oil, salt, and pepper)

Instructions:

1. In a bowl, combine cooked quinoa, mixed vegetables, herbs, and nuts.
2. Drizzle with lemon vinaigrette and toss to combine. Serve at room temperature.

Hummus and Veggie Wrap

Ingredients:

- Whole wheat tortilla or wrap
- Hummus
- Sliced cucumbers, bell peppers, tomatoes, and lettuce
- Olives (optional)
- Sprouts (optional)

Instructions:

1. Spread a generous amount of hummus on the tortilla.
2. Layer sliced vegetables, olives, and sprouts.
3. Roll up the tortilla, tucking in the sides as you go. Slice in half if desired.

Stuffed Bell Peppers

Ingredients:

- Bell peppers (any color)
- Cooked quinoa or rice
- Cooked black beans or lentils
- Diced tomatoes
- Chopped onion and garlic
- Ground cumin, paprika, and oregano
- Salt and pepper to taste

Instructions:

1. Preheat the oven to 375°F (190°C).
2. Cut the tops off bell peppers and remove seeds and membranes.
3. In a skillet, sauté onion and garlic until translucent. Add diced tomatoes, cooked quinoa or rice, cooked beans or lentils, and spices.
4. Stuff the bell peppers with the mixture and place them in a baking dish.

5. Bake for about 25-30 minutes, until the
   peppers are tender.

73

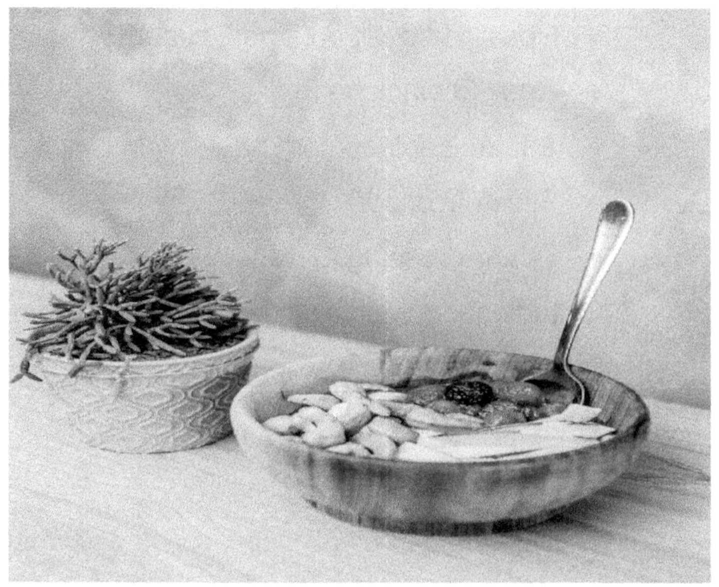

Sweet Potato and Black Bean Bowl

Ingredients:

- Roasted sweet potatoes, cubed
- Cooked black beans
- Sautéed spinach or kale
- Sliced avocado
- Tahini dressing (2 tablespoons tahini, 1 tablespoon lemon juice, water to thin, salt)

Instructions:

1. Assemble bowls with roasted sweet potatoes, black beans, sautéed greens, and avocado slices.
2. Drizzle with tahini dressing before serving.

Veggie Stir-Fry

Ingredients:

- Mixed stir-fry vegetables (broccoli, bell peppers, snap peas, carrots, etc.)
- Firm tofu, cubed
- Low-sodium soy sauce or teriyaki sauce
- Cooked brown rice or quinoa

Instructions:

1. In a wok or large skillet, sauté tofu until lightly browned. Remove from the pan.
2. Add mixed vegetables to the pan and stir-fry until tender-crisp.
3. Add tofu back to the pan and drizzle with soy sauce or teriyaki sauce. Toss to coat.
4. Serve over cooked brown rice or quinoa.

Spinach and Mushroom Pasta

Ingredients:

- Whole wheat pasta
- Fresh spinach
- Sliced mushrooms
- Chopped onion and garlic
- Olive oil
- Nutritional yeast (optional)
- Salt and pepper to taste

Instructions:

1. Cook pasta according to package instructions. Drain and set aside.
2. In a pan, sauté onion and garlic until fragrant. Add mushrooms and cook until browned.
3. Add fresh spinach and cook until wilted.
4. Toss cooked pasta with the vegetables, drizzle with olive oil, and season with nutritional yeast, salt, and pepper.

Mediterranean Wrap

Ingredients:

- Whole wheat tortilla or wrap
- Hummus
- Sliced cucumber, tomato, red onion
- Kalamata olives
- Fresh parsley
- Drizzle of balsamic vinegar

Instructions:

1. Spread hummus on the tortilla.
2. Layer cucumber, tomato, red onion, olives, and fresh parsley.
3. Drizzle with balsamic vinegar and wrap up the tortilla.

Vegetable and Lentil Curry

Ingredients:

- Cooked lentils (green or brown)
- Mixed vegetables (potatoes, carrots, peas, etc.)
- Chopped onion and garlic
- Curry powder, turmeric, cumin, and coriander
- Coconut milk
- Fresh cilantro (coriander) for garnish

Instructions:

1. In a pot, sauté onion and garlic until softened. Add curry powder, turmeric, cumin, and coriander.
2. Add mixed vegetables and cooked lentils. Pour in coconut milk and simmer until vegetables are tender.
3. Serve over cooked brown rice or quinoa. Garnish with fresh cilantro.

Chapter 5: Wholesome Dinners for Wellness

Vegetable Stir-Fry

Ingredients:

- Mixed stir-fry vegetables (broccoli, bell peppers, carrots, snap peas, etc.)
- Tofu or tempeh, cubed
- Low-sodium soy sauce or teriyaki sauce
- Cooked brown rice or quinoa

Instructions:

1. In a wok or large skillet, sauté tofu or tempeh until lightly browned. Remove from the pan.
2. Add mixed vegetables to the pan and stir-fry until tender-crisp.

3. Add tofu or tempeh back to the pan and
   drizzle with soy sauce or teriyaki sauce.
   Toss to coat.

4. Serve over cooked brown rice or quinoa.

Lentil Stew

Ingredients:

- 1 cup dried green or brown lentils
- 4 cups vegetable broth
- 1 onion, chopped
- 2 carrots, chopped
- 2 celery stalks, chopped
- 2 cloves garlic, minced
- 1 teaspoon thyme
- 1 bay leaf
- Salt and pepper to taste

Instructions:

1. Rinse lentils and set aside.
2. In a large pot, sauté onions, carrots, and celery until softened.
3. Add garlic, thyme, bay leaf, and lentils. Stir to combine.
4. Pour in vegetable broth, bring to a boil, then reduce heat and simmer for about 20-25 minutes until lentils are tender.

5. Season with salt and pepper. Remove the bay leaf before serving.

Roasted Vegetable Quinoa Bowl

Ingredients:

- Assorted roasted vegetables (sweet potatoes, Brussels sprouts, bell peppers, etc.)
- Cooked quinoa
- Chickpeas or beans
- Lemon tahini dressing (2 tablespoons tahini, 1 tablespoon lemon juice, water to thin, salt)

Instructions:

1. Arrange roasted vegetables, cooked quinoa, and chickpeas or beans in a bowl.
2. Drizzle with lemon tahini dressing before serving.

Baked Stuffed Bell Peppers

Ingredients:

- Bell peppers (any color)
- Cooked quinoa or rice
- Cooked black beans or lentils
- Diced tomatoes
- Chopped onion and garlic
- Ground cumin, paprika, and oregano
- Salt and pepper to taste

Instructions:

1. Preheat the oven to 375°F (190°C).
2. Cut the tops off bell peppers and remove seeds and membranes.
3. In a skillet, sauté onion and garlic until translucent. Add diced tomatoes, cooked quinoa or rice, cooked beans or lentils, and spices.
4. Stuff the bell peppers with the mixture and place them in a baking dish.

5. Bake for about 25-30 minutes, until the
    peppers are tender.

Vegan Chili

Ingredients:

- 1 can of cooked kidney beans or black beans, drained and rinsed
- 1 can of diced tomatoes
- 1 onion, chopped
- 1 red bell pepper, chopped
- 1 carrot, chopped
- 2 cloves garlic, minced
- 1 tablespoon chili powder
- 1 teaspoon cumin
- 1 teaspoon paprika
- Salt and pepper to taste

Instructions:

- In a large pot, sauté onion, bell pepper, and carrot until softened.
- Add minced garlic, chili powder, cumin, paprika, salt, and pepper. Stir for a minute.

- Add beans and diced tomatoes. Bring to a simmer and cook for about 20-25 minutes.
- Serve the chili hot with a side of whole grain bread or rice.

Mediterranean Quinoa Salad

Ingredients:

- Cooked quinoa
- Diced cucumber, tomato, red onion
- Chopped Kalamata olives
- Chopped fresh parsley
- Lemon vinaigrette (2 tablespoons lemon juice, 2 tablespoons olive oil, salt, and pepper)

Instructions:

1. In a bowl, combine cooked quinoa, diced vegetables, olives, and parsley.
2. Drizzle with lemon vinaigrette and toss to combine.

Vegan Lentil Shepherd's Pie

Ingredients:

- Cooked green or brown lentils
- Mixed vegetables (carrots, peas, corn)
- Mashed potatoes (made with plant-based milk and vegan butter)
- Nutritional yeast (optional)
- Salt and pepper to taste

Instructions:

1. Preheat the oven to 375°F (190°C).
2. In a baking dish, layer cooked lentils and mixed vegetables.
3. Spread mashed potatoes over the lentil mixture.
4. Bake for about 20-25 minutes, until the top is golden.
5. Sprinkle with nutritional yeast, salt, and pepper before serving.

Vegan Pasta Primavera

Ingredients:

- Whole wheat pasta
- Mixed sautéed vegetables (broccoli, bell peppers, zucchini, etc.)
- Cashew Alfredo sauce (blend soaked cashews, garlic, nutritional yeast, plant-based milk)
- Fresh basil or parsley for garnish

Instructions:

1. Cook pasta according to package instructions. Drain and set aside.
2. Sauté mixed vegetables until tender.
3. Blend soaked cashews, garlic, nutritional yeast, and plant-based milk to make the Alfredo sauce.
4. Toss cooked pasta, sautéed vegetables, and Alfredo sauce together.
5. Garnish with fresh basil or parsley before serving.

Chickpea and Spinach Curry

Ingredients:

- Cooked chickpeas
- Chopped onion and garlic
- Curry powder, cumin, coriander
- Diced tomatoes or tomato sauce
- Coconut milk
- Fresh spinach
- Lemon juice
- Salt and pepper to taste

Instructions:

1. In a pan, sauté onion and garlic until fragrant.
2. Add curry powder, cumin, and coriander. Stir for a minute.
3. Add cooked chickpeas and diced tomatoes or tomato sauce.

4. Pour in coconut milk and let it simmer
    for about 10 minutes.

5. Stir in fresh spinach until wilted. Add
    lemon juice, salt, and pepper.

Portobello Mushroom Steaks

Ingredients:

- Portobello mushroom caps
- Balsamic vinegar
- Olive oil
- Minced garlic
- Fresh rosemary or thyme
- Salt and pepper to taste

Instructions:

1. Preheat the oven to 400°F (200°C).
2. Mix balsamic vinegar, olive oil, minced garlic, chopped herbs, salt, and pepper in a bowl.
3. Brush the mushroom caps with the marinade on both sides.
4. Place the mushrooms on a baking sheet and bake for about 15-20 minutes, flipping once halfway through.
5. Serve the mushroom steaks with a side of roasted vegetables or a salad.

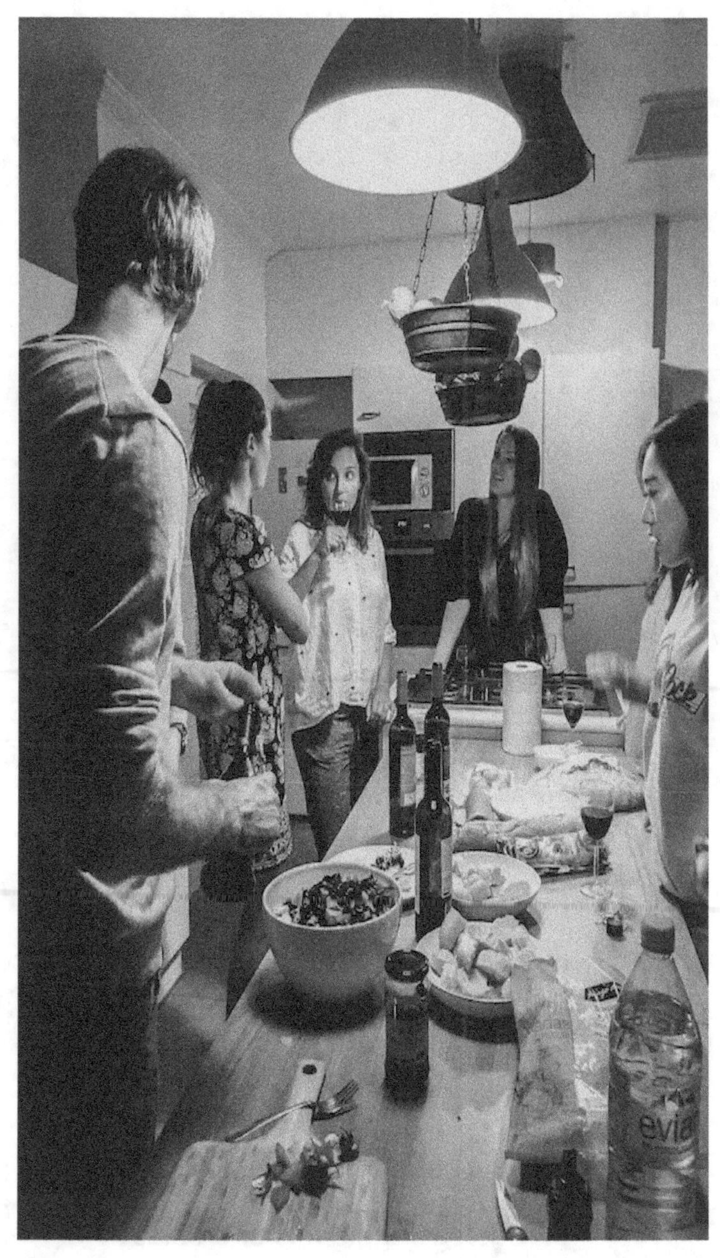

Chapter 6: Snacks and Appetizers

Hummus and Veggie Sticks

Ingredients:

- Hummus (store-bought or homemade)
- Sliced carrot sticks, cucumber, bell peppers, and celery

Instructions:

1. Arrange the sliced veggies on a plate.
2. Serve with a bowl of hummus for dipping.

Guacamole and Sliced Veggies

Ingredients:

- Ripe avocados
- Lime or lemon juice
- Diced tomatoes, red onion, cilantro
- Salt and pepper
- Sliced bell peppers, cucumber, and carrot sticks

Instructions:

1. Mash avocados and mix with lime or lemon juice, diced tomatoes, red onion, cilantro, salt, and pepper.
2. Serve with sliced veggies for dipping.

Rice Cakes with Nut Butter and Banana

Ingredients:

- Whole grain rice cakes
- Nut butter (almond, peanut, or cashew)
- Sliced banana

Instructions:

1. Spread nut butter on rice cakes.
2. Top with sliced banana.

Trail Mix

Ingredients:

- Nuts (almonds, walnuts, cashews)
- Seeds (pumpkin seeds, sunflower seeds)
- Dried fruits (raisins, cranberries, apricots)

Instructions:

1. Mix together nuts, seeds, and dried fruits in a bowl.
2. Portion into small snack-sized bags for easy grab-and-go.

Greek Salad Skewers

Ingredients:

- Cherry tomatoes
- Cucumber chunks
- Kalamata olives
- Vegan feta cheese (optional)
- Fresh basil leaves

Instructions:

1. Thread cherry tomatoes, cucumber chunks, olives, and vegan feta onto small skewers.
2. Garnish with fresh basil leaves.

Sliced Apple with Nut Butter

Ingredients:

- Sliced apples
- Nut butter (almond, peanut, or cashew)

Instructions:

1. Spread nut butter on apple slices.

Roasted Chickpeas

Ingredients:

- Cooked chickpeas
- Olive oil
- Spices (paprika, cumin, garlic powder)
- Salt and pepper

Instructions:

1. Preheat the oven to 400°F (200°C).
2. Toss cooked chickpeas with olive oil, spices, salt, and pepper.
3. Roast in the oven for about 20-25 minutes until crispy.

Veggie Spring Rolls

Ingredients:

- Rice paper wrappers
- Sliced vegetables (bell peppers, carrots, cucumber, lettuce)
- Fresh herbs (mint, basil, cilantro)
- Dipping sauce (peanut sauce or soy-based sauce)

Instructions:

1. Dip rice paper wrappers in warm water to soften.
2. Fill with sliced vegetables and fresh herbs.
3. Roll up tightly and serve with dipping sauce.

Cucumber Bites with Hummus

Ingredients:

- Sliced cucumber rounds
- Hummus
- Chopped fresh dill (optional)

Instructions:

1. Spread a small amount of hummus on each cucumber round.
2. Garnish with chopped fresh dill if desired.

Fruit Salad Cups

Ingredients:

- Assorted fresh fruits (berries, melon, grapes, kiwi, etc.)
- Fresh mint leaves

Instructions:

1. Wash, peel, and chop fruits into small pieces.
2. Arrange in small serving cups and garnish with fresh mint leaves.

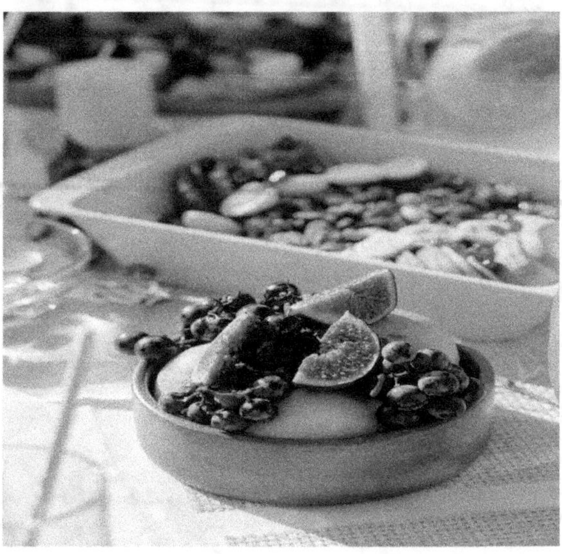

Chapter 7: Desserts

Fruit Salad

Ingredients:

- Assorted fresh fruits (berries, melon, grapes, kiwi, etc.)
- Fresh mint leaves

Instructions:

1. Wash, peel, and chop fruits into bite-sized pieces.
2. Combine the fruits in a bowl and garnish with fresh mint leaves.

Banana "Nice Cream"

Ingredients:

- Ripe bananas, sliced and frozen
- Plant-based milk (if needed)
- Toppings: chopped nuts, shredded coconut, dark chocolate chips

Instructions:

1. Blend frozen banana slices in a food processor until smooth and creamy. Add a splash of plant-based milk if necessary.
2. Serve in bowls and top with your favorite toppings.

Baked Apples

Ingredients:

- Apples, cored
- Cinnamon
- Chopped nuts
- Maple syrup (optional)

Instructions:

1. Preheat the oven to 350°F (175°C).
2. Sprinkle cinnamon and chopped nuts into the cored apples.
3. Place apples in a baking dish and drizzle with maple syrup if desired.
4. Bake for about 20-25 minutes until the apples are soft.

Chia Seed Pudding

Ingredients:

- Chia seeds
- Plant-based milk
- Vanilla extract
- Fresh fruits or berries

Instructions:

1. Mix chia seeds, plant-based milk, and vanilla extract in a bowl.
2. Stir well and let it sit in the refrigerator for at least 2 hours or overnight.
3. Top with fresh fruits or berries before serving.

Coconut Yogurt Parfait

Ingredients:

- Plant-based coconut yogurt
- Mixed berries
- Granola
- Drizzle of agave syrup

Instructions:

1. Layer coconut yogurt, mixed berries, and granola in a glass or bowl.
2. Drizzle with agave syrup for added sweetness.

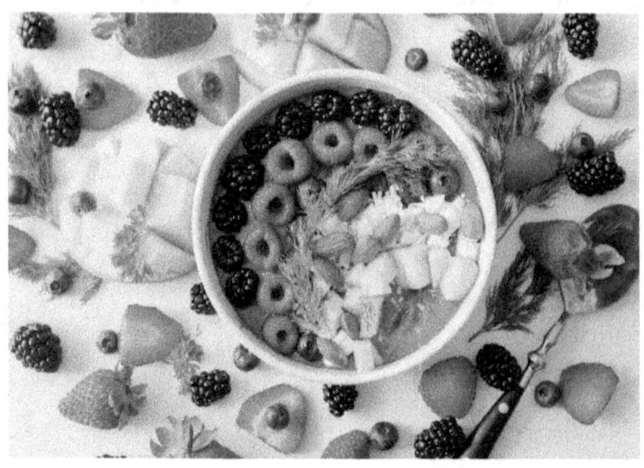

Vegan Chocolate Pudding

Ingredients:

- Ripe avocados
- Cocoa powder
- Plant-based milk
- Sweetener (agave syrup, maple syrup)
- Vanilla extract

Instructions:

1. Blend avocados, cocoa powder, plant-based milk, sweetener, and vanilla extract until smooth and creamy.
2. Chill in the refrigerator before serving.

Rice Pudding

Ingredients:

- Cooked rice (white or brown)
- Plant-based milk
- Sweetener (agave syrup, maple syrup)
- Ground cinnamon
- Raisins or dried fruits (optional)

Instructions:

1. In a saucepan, combine cooked rice, plant-based milk, sweetener, and ground cinnamon.
2. Cook over low heat, stirring frequently, until the mixture thickens.
3. Stir in raisins or dried fruits if using. Serve warm or chilled.

Oatmeal Cookies

Ingredients:

- Rolled oats
- Mashed bananas
- Raisins or chopped dates
- Cinnamon
- Vanilla extract

Instructions:

1. Preheat the oven to 350°F (175°C).
2. Mix rolled oats, mashed bananas, raisins or dates, cinnamon, and vanilla extract in a bowl.
3. Drop spoonfuls of the mixture onto a baking sheet and flatten with a fork.
4. Bake for about 15-20 minutes until golden brown.

Mixed Berry Crumble

Ingredients:

- Mixed berries (blueberries, strawberries, raspberries)
- Rolled oats
- Almond flour or whole wheat flour
- Coconut oil
- Maple syrup

Instructions:

1. Preheat the oven to 375°F (190°C).
2. Place mixed berries in a baking dish.
3. In a bowl, mix rolled oats, almond flour or whole wheat flour, coconut oil, and maple syrup to create a crumble topping.
4. Spread the crumble over the berries and bake for about 25-30 minutes until bubbly and golden.

Chocolate-Dipped Strawberries

Ingredients:

- Fresh strawberries
- Dark chocolate chips or vegan chocolate
- Chopped nuts or coconut flakes (optional)

Instructions:

1. Melt dark chocolate chips in a microwave or over a double boiler.
2. Dip each strawberry into the melted chocolate, allowing excess to drip off.
3. Place the chocolate-dipped strawberries on a parchment-lined tray.
4. Sprinkle with chopped nuts or coconut flakes if desired.
5. Let them cool and harden in the refrigerator before serving.

BONUS: Tips for a Holistic and Healthy Lifestyle

A plant-based lifestyle extends beyond the food we eat—it encompasses our overall well-being. In this chapter of the "Plant-Based Diet Cookbook for Elders," we explore Tips for a Holistic and Healthy Lifestyle. From cultivating mindfulness to embracing physical activity, these insights guide you in creating a life that harmoniously integrates nourishment, vitality, and purpose.

Embracing Holistic Wellness

Holistic well-being embraces the interconnectedness of physical, mental, emotional, and spiritual aspects of life.

Prioritizing Mindful Eating

1. **Savoring Each Bite:** Practice mindful eating by savoring flavors, textures, and aromas, fostering a deeper connection with your meals.

2. **Eating with Gratitude:** Cultivate gratitude for the nourishment you receive from plant-based foods, enhancing the enjoyment of your meals.

Engaging in Regular Physical Activity

1. **Age-Appropriate Activities:** Participate in physical activities that align with your abilities, whether it's gentle yoga, walking, swimming, or dancing.

2. **Functional Fitness:** Focus on exercises that improve mobility, balance,

and flexibility, enhancing your quality of life.

Nurturing Mental and Emotional Health

1. **Mindfulness Practices:** Explore meditation, deep breathing, and mindfulness techniques to reduce stress and promote emotional well-being.
2. **Creative Outlets:** Engage in hobbies or creative pursuits that bring joy and contribute to mental clarity.

Connecting with Nature

1. **Outdoor Exploration:** Spend time outdoors, whether it's gardening, hiking, or simply enjoying the beauty of natural surroundings.
2. **Vitamin D Absorption:** Sunlight exposure supports vitamin D synthesis, benefiting bone health and mood regulation.

Cultivating Meaningful Relationships

1. **Social Connections:** Foster relationships with friends, family, and community members that promote a sense of belonging and support.
2. **Acts of Kindness:** Engage in acts of kindness and volunteerism, contributing to a sense of purpose and well-being.

Prioritizing Sleep and Rest

1. **Sleep Hygiene:** Establish a calming bedtime routine and create a sleep-conducive environment for restorative sleep.
2. **Napping:** Incorporate short naps to recharge during the day and enhance cognitive function.

Reducing Stress and Relaxation

1. **Stress-Relief Techniques:** Practice stress-relief techniques such as

meditation, progressive muscle relaxation, or aromatherapy.

2. **Relaxation Rituals:** Develop relaxation rituals, such as taking warm baths, reading, or practicing gentle stretching.

Celebrating Self-Care

1. **Treating Yourself:** Embrace self-care practices such as spa treatments, self-massage, or enjoying a favorite book or movie.
2. **Unplugging:** Disconnect from electronic devices periodically to create mental space and promote relaxation.

Beyond the Plate: Incorporating Mindfulness and Wellness

A plant-based lifestyle extends beyond the food we consume; it encompasses the way we approach life as a whole. In this sub-chapter of the "Plant-Based Diet Cookbook for Elders," we delve into the realm of Beyond the Plate: Incorporating Mindfulness and Wellness. These insights guide you in embracing a mindful and holistic approach to nourishing not just your body, but also your mind and soul.

The Power of Mindful Living

Mindfulness is the practice of being present in the moment, cultivating awareness, and nurturing a deeper connection to your surroundings and yourself.

Mindful Eating for Nourishment

1. **Savoring Flavors:** Engage your senses in the act of eating, paying attention to the flavors, textures, and aromas of your meals.

2. **Eating with Intention:** Approach each meal with gratitude and intention, acknowledging the nourishment you're providing to your body.

Mindful Movement and Physical Activity

1. **Conscious Exercise:** Engage in physical activities with mindfulness, focusing on how your body moves and the sensations you experience.

2. **Connecting with Breath:** Incorporate mindful breathing techniques into your workouts to enhance relaxation and energy flow.

Mindful Moments for Relaxation

1. **Mindful Breathing:** Dedicate moments throughout the day to focus on your breath, inhaling calmness and exhaling tension.

2. **Mindful Walking:** Practice walking mindfully, being fully present with each step and the sensations in your body.

Mindfulness for Emotional Well-Being

1. **Emotional Awareness:** Cultivate an awareness of your emotions without judgment, allowing yourself to feel and process them.

2. **Mindful Responses:** Respond to emotions with mindfulness, choosing conscious actions that align with your well-being.

Cultivating Gratitude and Joy

1. **Daily Reflection:** Take time each day to reflect on moments of gratitude and joy, regardless of their size.
2. **Mindful Moments of Joy:** Engage in activities that bring you joy, whether it's reading, spending time with loved ones, or pursuing hobbies.

Mindfulness Rituals

1. **Morning Ritual:** Begin your day with a mindful moment, setting positive intentions for the hours ahead.
2. **Evening Reflection:** Wind down with a reflective practice, expressing gratitude for the day's experiences.

Mindfulness in Social Interactions

1. **Active Listening:** Engage in active listening during conversations, fully immersing yourself in the present moment.

2. **Empathy and Compassion:** Approach interactions with empathy and compassion, creating meaningful connections.

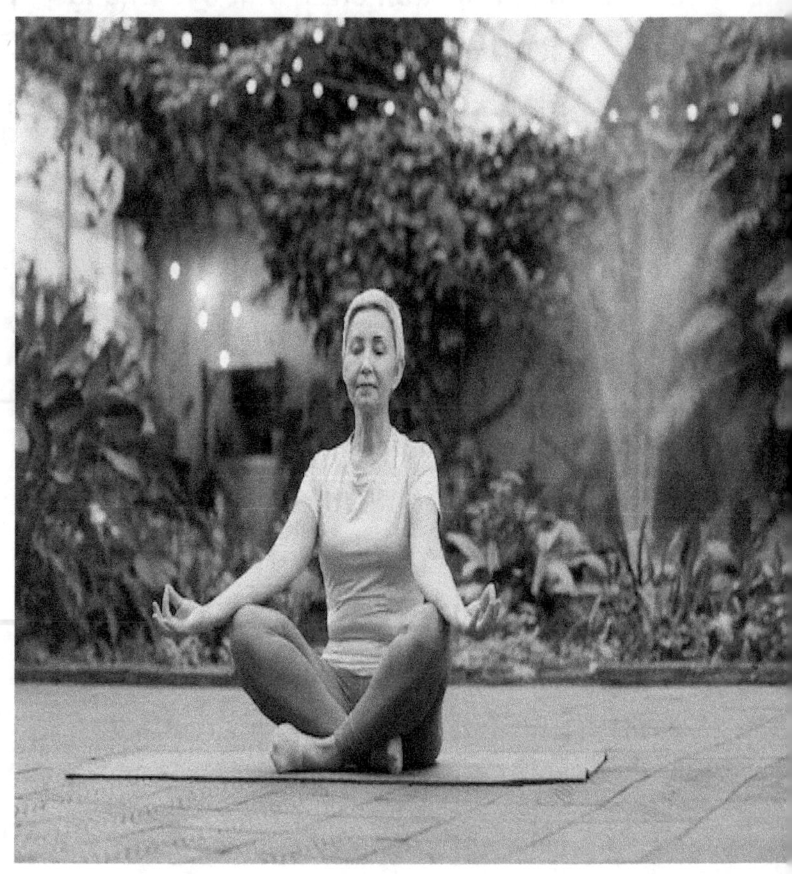

Staying Active, Managing Stress, and Getting Quality Sleep

A harmonious life is achieved by nurturing the interplay of physical activity, stress management, and restful sleep. In this sub-chapter of the "Plant-Based Diet Cookbook for Elders," we explore the synergy of Staying Active, Managing Stress, and Getting Quality Sleep. These insights guide you in fostering a balanced and holistic approach to well-being, enhancing your plant-based journey and overall vitality.

The Holistic Connection

The triad of staying active, managing stress, and getting quality sleep forms the cornerstone of holistic well-being, benefiting every aspect of your life.

Staying Active

1. **Finding Joy in Movement:** Engage in activities you enjoy, whether it's walking, gardening, dancing, or yoga, promoting a lifelong commitment to physical well-being.

2. **Functional Fitness:** Focus on exercises that improve balance, flexibility, and mobility, enhancing your ability to carry out daily activities.

3. **Social Engagement:** Participate in group activities or classes, fostering social connections while nurturing your physical health.

Managing Stress

1. **Mindfulness Practices:** Incorporate mindfulness meditation, deep breathing, and progressive muscle relaxation to manage stress and promote emotional well-being.

2. **Nature Connection:** Spend time in nature, allowing the serenity of the outdoors to alleviate stress and restore mental clarity.

3. **Creative Outlets:** Engage in creative activities such as painting, writing, or playing music, providing an outlet for self-expression and stress relief.

Getting Quality Sleep

1. **Sleep Hygiene:** Establish a soothing bedtime routine, creating an environment conducive to restful sleep.

2. **Regular Schedule:** Maintain consistent sleep and wake times to regulate your body's internal clock and enhance sleep quality.

3. **Unplugging:** Reduce screen time before bed to promote relaxation and improve sleep onset.

Mind-Body Connection

1. **Mindful Movement:** Integrate mindfulness into your physical activities, aligning your body and mind for enhanced well-being.

2. **Stress-Aware Exercise:** Engage in stress-reducing exercises like tai chi or gentle yoga, focusing on the mind-body connection.

Prioritizing Self-Care

1. **Scheduled Me-Time:** Dedicate time each day for self-care activities, whether it's reading, taking a bath, or enjoying a favorite hobby.

2. **Healthy Boundaries:** Set boundaries to avoid overcommitment and create space for self-nurturing activities.

Conclusion

As we bring our journey through the "Plant-Based Diet Cookbook for Elders" to a close, we reflect on the remarkable tapestry of health, flavors, and vitality that we have woven together. This cookbook is more than just a collection of recipes; it's a celebration of the profound impact that plant-based choices can have on our well-being and the world around us.

Throughout these pages, we have explored the colorful world of plant-based cuisine, from energizing breakfasts to wholesome dinners, from guilt-free desserts to mindful snacking. We've discovered that embracing a plant-based lifestyle is not only about what we eat but also about nurturing our bodies, minds, and spirits in a holistic way.

In our journey, we've learned the art of crafting nutrient-rich meals that invigorate our bodies with essential vitamins, minerals, and antioxidants. We've uncovered the joy of exploring diverse flavors and ingredients that reflect the richness of nature's bounty. More than that, we've discovered that each meal is an opportunity to show gratitude for the nourishment we receive and to cultivate a deeper connection with the Earth and its creatures.

But this cookbook is not just about recipes; it's about fostering mindfulness and cultivating well-being. It's about recognizing that our choices ripple beyond our plates, affecting our physical health, emotional balance, and ethical compass. We've explored the power of mindful eating, the beauty of incorporating movement and relaxation, and the significance of connecting with our communities and the world at large.

As we close this chapter, let us carry the wisdom and inspiration of these pages into our lives. May the recipes you've discovered and the insights you've gained empower you to embrace a lifestyle that resonates with vibrant health, compassion, and purpose. Let this cookbook be a trusted companion on your journey to greater well-being, offering nourishment not only to your body but also to your heart and soul.

Thank you for embarking on this plant-based adventure with us. May your path be filled with delicious meals, joyful moments, and the fulfillment that comes from nurturing yourself, those around you, and the planet we all call home. Remember, with every bite you take, you're choosing a life of vitality, harmony, and the profound beauty of living in alignment with your values. Here's to the joy of a plant-based journey that nourishes not just your body, but your entire being.